High Fiber Keto For Women

A Beginner's 5-Step Guide, With Sample Recipes and a 7-Day Meal Plan

Disclaimer

By reading this disclaimer, you are accepting the terms of the disclaimer in full. If you disagree with this disclaimer, please do not read the guide.

All of the content within this guide is provided for informational and educational purposes only, and should not be accepted as independent medical or other professional advice. The author is not a doctor, physician, nurse, mental health provider, or registered nutritionist/dietician. Therefore, using and reading this guide does not establish any form of a physician-patient relationship.

Always consult with a physician or another qualified health provider with any issues or questions you might have regarding any sort of medical condition. Do not ever disregard any qualified professional medical advice or delay seeking that advice because of anything you have read in this guide. The information in this guide is not intended to be any sort of medical advice and should not be used in lieu of any medical advice by a licensed and qualified medical professional.

Where applicable, persons shown in the cover images are stock photography models and the publisher has obtained the rights to use the images through license agreements with third-party stock image companies.

Table of Contents

Introduction

Do you ever wish to eat healthy and lessen your cravings for unhealthy foods? Are you in search of a healthy diet that suits your lifestyle, health goals, and preferences? The high-fiber ketogenic diet is what you might have been looking for!

Known for its mental health benefits and overall well-being, the ketogenic diet is now a popular, sought-after kind of diet for health advocates. It features a high-fat, low-carb meal structure that will help in weight loss, managing sugar in the blood, managing hormonal imbalance, and improving neurological health.

Imagine reaping these benefits but with bonuses including a healthy gut microbiota and healthy skin. This is how fiber enhances the benefits of the ketogenic diet.

In this comprehensive guide, we'll walk you through these topics regarding the high-fiber ketogenic diet:

• What is a ketogenic diet, its basic principles and components, and its history?
• How does the ketogenic work in the body?

- What are the types of ketogenic diet and which one is suitable for you?
- Adding fiber to the ketogenic diet.
- Types of fiber and a 5-step guide on how to incorporate fiber into the ketogenic diet.
- What are the health benefits of a high-fiber ketogenic diet?
- Women and the high-fiber ketogenic diet relationship.
- Sample recipes of high-fiber ketogenic diet meals.

Keep reading for rich information about this packed with the benefits of a high-fiber ketogenic diet.

What Is the Ketogenic Diet?

In this section, we'll talk about the key concepts, history, origin, and variations of the Ketogenic diet so we'll better understand what it is.

The ketogenic diet is a low-carb, high-fat eating structure plan that will force the body to achieve ketosis.

As we know, our body uses energy in the form of calories. For the most common diet, the main source of calories is carbohydrates like rice, pasta, and bread. But with the Ketogenic diet, where more fat is ingested than carbs, the body will be forced to burn the fats to be used for energy instead of the carbs because of their low availability. This metabolic state is called ketosis.

The body achieves ketosis by breaking down the fats from the food intake and the body's stored fats into ketones which can be used as a source of energy, especially for the brain.

The Fundamentals of the Ketogenic Diet

Ketosis and macronutrient distribution (high-fat, moderate protein, low-carb) are closely related as they are fundamental components of the ketogenic diet.

A ketogenic diet usually implies that around 70-75% of the caloric intake comes from fat, protein contributes about 20-25% and just a small portion, 5-10%, is derived from carbohydrates. This specific distribution is designed to push the body into a metabolic state known as ketosis.

In ketosis, due to the scarcity of carbohydrates (which are usually the body's primary source of energy), the body starts to burn fat for energy instead. It does this by breaking down dietary and stored fat into molecules called ketones, which can be used as a source of energy, especially for the brain.

So, a high fat intake is necessary to provide enough fuel for the body, a moderate protein intake ensures muscle mass is maintained, and a low carbohydrate intake is critical for maintaining the state of ketosis.

Therefore, achieving and maintaining ketosis in a ketogenic diet heavily relies on adhering to this specific macronutrient distribution. We'll discuss this in further detail in the following sections.

History and Origin of the Ketogenic Diet

In ancient times, fasting was used as a method to prevent seizures. It has been recognized and widely used by the ancient Greeks.

In the early 1920s and 1930s, the Ketogenic diet became popular in treating epilepsy. This is to mimic the benefits of fasting while still providing nutrition. However, when anticonvulsant drugs were introduced in the early 1940s, the Ketogenic diet became unpopular and is fated to be forgotten.

Although it was believed that the anticonvulsant medication could treat and subsequently eliminate epilepsy, it was later revealed that there were drug-resistant epileptic patients. And so, in the 1990s, the Ketogenic diet made a comeback to treat those drug-resistant epilepsy in children.

Over time, the Ketogenic diet's potential benefits for weight loss have been recognized. It was widely used beyond the treatment of epilepsy but also for the management of diabetes and overall well-being. It transitioned from a medically supervised diet to a popular lifestyle choice.

Fast forward to the 21st century, the Ketogenic Diet has drawn the interest of researchers, exploring more of its health benefits including the management of Alzheimer's disease, metabolic syndrome, and cancer treatment.

In recent years, it gained popularity as more celebrities and influencers have vouched for this diet and claimed that it helped them lose weight and improved their well-being. There are now emerging variations of this diet that we will discuss in the next chapters.

Variations of the Ketogenic Diet

Why are there Ketogenic Diet variations?

Standard Ketogenic Diet

The Standard Ketogenic diet comprises 70-75% of calories from fat, 20-25% from protein, and only 5-10% from carbohydrates and this seems to be restrictive and challenging in terms of food options. While the Standard Ketogenic Diet may work for some, it is not for everyone.

This is why there are now variations of the Ketogenic diet that will cater to the individual's needs, preferences, and lifestyle.

High-Protein Ketogenic Diet

For those who are into bodybuilding, the most suitable Ketogenic diet would be the High-Protein Ketogenic Diet. This Ketogenic Diet variation has a macronutrient ratio of 60% fat, 35% protein, and 5% carbs.

Targeted Ketogenic Diet

If you're an athlete or into high-intensity physical activity, the Targeted Ketogenic Diet may be best for you. This Ketogenic Diet variation is very similar to the Standard Ketogenic diet in terms of macronutrient ratio except that it allows you to eat additional carbs around your workout times. Depending on the intensity of the physical activity, you can consume 20-50 grams of additional carbs 30 minutes to 1 hour before your exercise.

Cyclical Ketogenic Diet

On the other hand, the Cyclical Ketogenic Diet offers an easy-to-follow structure for the long term as it gives you breaks from consuming low-carb. This variation will give you periods of high-carb refeeds such as 5 ketogenic days followed by 2 high-carb days. Though this ketogenic variation is easy to adhere to, it demands stringent monitoring to make sure you return to the state of ketosis after consuming a high amount of carbs.

Through these variations, individuals are given the chance to choose the best option that suits their preferences, lifestyle, and health objectives.

And there you have it. Hope you have now gained a better understanding of the Ketogenic diet, its origin, key concepts, and variations. But the learning doesn't end here because we'll embark on a deeper detail about this controversial diet.

In the following sections, we'll delve into the principles of this diet and how to make it worth it.

Basic principles and components of a Ketogenic diet

Now that you've gained a better understanding of what a Ketogenic diet is, let's discuss its basic principles and concepts.

Basic Principles of the Ketogenic Diet

As we have previously discussed, the Ketogenic diet revolves around the high-fat, low-carb eating structure to achieve ketosis. We've also touched points about the macronutrient ratios for the Ketogenic Diet variations which include the carbon, fat, and protein intake. But how would you utilize this information to make this diet effective?

Components of the Ketogenic Diet

To make the Ketogenic Diet effective, we need to understand the importance of each macronutrient.

High-Fat Intake: In the ketogenic diet, fat must take up most of your meal, around 70-75%. It is where most of your caloric intake must come from to encourage your body to use your fat for energy instead of glucose from carbohydrates. However, it is crucial to be mindful about your choices of fatty foods. It is best that you stick with healthy fats including avocado, salmon, olive oil, and nuts.

Low-Carb: The Ketogenic diet significantly limits carbohydrate intake, usually to around 5-10% of your daily calories. This low-carb intake is crucial to maintain the state of ketosis. When your carbohydrate intake is low, your body depletes its stored glucose and starts breaking down fat for energy. Low-carb vegetables, nuts, and dairy products are good sources of carbohydrates for this diet.

Protein: Protein is vital for muscle growth. Common sources of protein are meat, fish, eggs, and tofu. For your protein consumption in the ketogenic diet, you must limit your intake. Protein should usually take up 20-25% of your daily calories. Consuming beyond this range will hinder ketosis from happening. This is because proteins are amino acids and excess amino acids in the system will be converted to glucose which is an energy source. So, instead of consuming your body's stored fats for energy, this excess glucose will be used as an energy source.

Fiber: Another macronutrient to consider in the ketogenic diet is fiber. While fat, carbohydrates, and proteins are the primary macronutrients in the ketogenic diet, fiber also plays a crucial role. Incorporating fiber into your meal will make you feel full thus keeping you from overfeeding or wanting to eat more. Common sources of fiber are leafy greens, broccoli, avocado, berries, nuts, and seeds. We'll elaborate more on this macronutrient in the following chapters.

By gaining insights into these macronutrients, you're on your way to choosing the right ketogenic diet variations that will suit your lifestyle, health goals, and personal preferences.

Importance of Hydration and Electrolytes

When following the ketogenic diet it is important to increase the intake of water. This is because the process of burning fats requires water molecules and the ketogenic diet may lead to greater fluid excretion. Also drinking more water while on the ketogenic diet can help weight loss to take a faster effect. This is because all macronutrients require water for metabolism.

Maintaining electrolyte balance is also important in the ketogenic diet as it helps in preventing symptoms like keto flu, supports heart and muscle functions, ensures neurological operation and digestion, and regulates fluid balance. Electrolytes such as sodium, potassium, calcium, magnesium, and chloride are essential minerals that play significant roles in various body functions.

Overall when following a ketogenic diet it is essential to drink more water to maintain the electrolyte balance. Always listen to your body's signal and drink when you are thirsty. To maintain proper electrolyte balance while following a ketogenic diet incorporating certain foods and supplements into your diet may be necessary. We will discuss some supplements that support the keto diet in the next section.

Potential Supplements for a Ketogenic Diet

As we have mentioned, incorporating certain foods and supplements into your meals when following a ketogenic diet may be necessary. While adhering to the diet alone will provide you with the necessary nutrients, taking supplements may help to manage the side effects of the diet or accelerate the benefits of the diet. Take a look at this compilation of supplements that you might want to add to your ketogenic meals.

MCT Oil

Incorporating Medium Chain Triglycerides or MCT oil into your ketogenic diet can enhance its benefits. MCT oil is a unique fat that is absorbed easily and quickly by the body. Once they are absorbed, they go directly straight to the liver where they are converted into ketones essential to reach the state of ketosis. We'll talk in deeper detail about how the body works during this process in the following chapters. But for now, think of MCT oil as a supplement essential for achieving ketosis faster.

There are several ways to incorporate MCT oil into your diet and these ways are pretty straightforward. You can either add them to your food or drinks. Whether you drizzle some to your salad, add them to your smoothie or coffee, or use it as a cooking oil, this supplement is an easy addition to your ketogenic diet.

Exogenous Ketones

These are ketones that are consumed through nutritional supplements, rather than produced in the body. They can provide enough sources of ketones whether you're in the state of ketosis or not. This can be useful to those who want to get ketosis's benefits without following the diet strictly.

Exogenous Ketones are available in the market in various forms. They can be in the form of salt including potassium, calcium, sodium, or magnesium. They are usually in powder form or encapsulated. The other form of exogenous ketones is the esters. Esters are raw ketones and are often associated with strong and undesirable taste. However, they are more effective in raising the ketone in the blood compared to salts. Esters are usually bought in liquid form but they are also available in powder and oil.

Omega-3 Fatty Acids

Omega-3 fatty acids are a type of polyunsaturated fat that is essential for overall health. They play a crucial role in numerous bodily functions, including heart health, brain function, mood regulation, and inflammation control. There are 3 main types of Omega-3 fatty acids - ALA which is plant-based omega-3 fatty acids found in chia seeds, walnuts, hemp seeds, and flaxseeds, EPA and DHA which can be found in fatty fish like salmon, fish oils, and algae supplements.

In the context of a ketogenic diet, Omega-3 fatty acids are especially important. A well-formulated ketogenic diet should be high in quality fats, and incorporating Omega-3s can help ensure that you're getting a balance of different fats. Additionally, Omega-3s can contribute to maintaining a state of ketosis because they are not easily stored as body fat and do not promote insulin resistance.

Vitamin and Mineral Supplements

When you're following a ketogenic diet, chances are, you'll skip some essential vitamins and minerals that are essential for your overall well-being. This is because, in the ketogenic diet, you have limited choices of food. So, adding vitamins and mineral supplements while on the ketogenic diet is crucial. Here are the key vitamins and minerals that you might want to consider while in the ketogenic diet:

Vitamin D: While our body can produce Vitamin D naturally through sun exposure, there will be times when we don't get enough. This is significantly true for people living in a country where sunlight is limited. Vitamin D is an essential vitamin that helps us with our immune function, bone health, and mood regulation. Adding this vitamin to your ketogenic diet will ensure you get enough vitamin D despite following a restrictive diet.

B Vitamins: While many foods in the ketogenic diet are rich in B vitamins such as eggs and meat, some advocates and aspirants of this diet are vegan. If you're one of them, you must get enough B vitamins, and another way to achieve this is through supplementation. B vitamins are essential in brain function, energy production, and cell metabolism.

Zinc: Zinc plays an important role in wound healing, the immune system, protein, and DNA synthesis. This mineral can be usually acquired from meat, shellfish, legumes, and seeds. However, if you're a vegan, pregnant woman, with a digestive disorder, or alcoholic you might need more zinc sources other than your daily food intake.

Remember, while these supplements can help fill nutritional gaps, they should not replace a balanced diet. It's always best to aim to get as many nutrients as possible from whole food sources and use supplements as an adjunct to a healthy diet. Also, it's crucial to consult with a healthcare professional before starting any new supplement regimen.

Now that we have touched points with the principles and components of the ketogenic diet, let's delve into the science of this diet including how it works in the body.

How the Ketogenic Diet Works in the Body

In this chapter, we will talk about how the ketogenic works in the body. We will explore the metabolic state of ketosis, the shift from glucose to fat for energy, the role of insulin and other hormones, the impact on brain function, and the long-term effects of the ketogenic diet on the body.

Metabolic State of Ketosis

As previously discussed in Chapter 2, ketosis is a metabolic state that takes place when the body's primary energy fuel which is carbohydrates is depleted forcing the body to utilize its stored fats for energy. The liver plays an important role in ketosis. When your carbohydrates are low, your insulin levels will also plummet. This will signal the liver to start breaking down stored fats or fats from your diet initially through the digestive system. This will convert the fats into fatty acids which are then transported to the liver.

In the liver, these fatty acids are converted into ketone bodies (or ketones) through a process called ketogenesis. The ketones are then released into the bloodstream, where they can be used by various tissues and organs, including the brain, as a source of energy.

The Role of Ketones in The Body

Ketones are crucial as the body's alternative energy source when glucose is at its lowest level during the ketogenic diet.

When carbohydrates are limited, the body's glucose becomes depleted. As a result, insulin levels decrease, signaling the liver to start breaking down stored fat into fatty acids. These fatty acids are then converted into ketone bodies through a process called ketogenesis.

During the metabolic state of ketosis, our brain heavily relies on ketones as its energy source. Unlike any other cells in our bodies, the brain cells called neurons can not immediately absorb fatty acids. Ketones, on the other hand, can cross the blood-brain barrier and provide the necessary fuel for the brain. In fact, during periods of sustained low carbohydrate intake, ketones can supply up to 70% of the brain's energy needs.

This just goes to show the many wonders of how our body adapts to changes and takes on survival mode in times when food supply is a challenge.

The Shift from Glucose to Fat for Energy

Glucose is a simple form of sugar derived from the carbohydrates that we eat including rice, pasta, bread, fruits, and vegetables. Simply put, glucose is the cells' food that gives them the energy to do their tasks.

However, glucose can't enter the cells on its own. This is where the insulin from your pancreas comes into play. Insulin is a hormone generally produced by the pancreas mostly after eating. Its task is to signal the cells to take in glucose, like a key that opens the cell doors for the glucose to come in.

This is when the process called glycolysis takes place. After entering the cell's cytoplasm, glucose is then broken down into molecules to generate energy in the form of Adenosine Triphosphate or ATP. ATP is often referred to as the cell's energy "currency". When you're carrying out work, your cells are "spending" ATP in exchange for energy.

When there are extra ATPs, your cells convert them into glycogen and store them in your liver for later use. When blood glucose levels decrease, another hormone called glucagon signals the breakdown of glycogen back into glucose to be released into the bloodstream, ensuring that the body has a constant supply of energy.

The Role of Insulin and Other Hormones

As has been previously discussed, insulin is a hormone stored in the pancreas that helps the cells to take in glucose and convert it to energy called ATP. In the state where there is extra glucose in your bloodstream, probably after overeating, your pancreas releases more insulin. The insulin converts glucose into glycogen, which is then stored in the liver for later use as an energy source when blood glucose levels are low.

Releasing more insulin over a long period will lead to insulin resistance. This is when insulin is not as effective in helping the cells to take in glucose which will result in high levels of glucose in your bloodstream. This often leads to Type 2 Diabetes, creating a vicious cycle wherein your pancreas keeps releasing more insulin.

This is where the ketogenic diet plays a significant role in reversing this state. As you already know, the ketogenic diet requires significantly low-carbohydrate intake. This will help control the pancreas in releasing insulin into your bloodstream since glucose is reduced when you eat fewer carbs. Also, your cell sensitivity to insulin will be restored which means they will take in glucose more effectively leading to maintaining blood sugar levels.

Ghrelin and Leptin

These two hormones are the opposite of each other as they are responsible for hunger and satiety. Ghrelin is produced in the stomach and its role is to stimulate appetite and promote fat storage. On the other hand, Leptin is produced by the fat cells and sends signals to the brain to inhibit hunger when adequate energy has been stored.

The high-fat, low-fat eating structure of the ketogenic diet has been linked to the decrease of Ghrelin hormones, thereby reducing the sensation of hunger. This is because dietary fats take more time to be digested compared to carbohydrates.

On the other hand, it is thought that following a ketogenic diet can either increase or decrease one's sensitivity to Leptin. Some studies suggest that your sensitivity to Leptin increases when following a ketogenic diet, making you more satisfied. On the contrary, some researchers suggested that the long-term use of a ketogenic diet can increase your resistance to Leptin because of the high-fat intake diet. These points still need more research though to prove the ketogenic diet's effect on these hormones.

Other Hormonal Changes

The ketogenic diet can indeed affect your insulin, ghrelin, and leptin hormones. Another hormone that may be affected by the ketogenic diet is cortisol. The cortisol hormone is responsible for various bodily functions including managing how your body uses carbohydrates, fats, and proteins, and helps your body respond to stress.

When you first start a ketogenic diet, your body has to adjust to using fat for fuel instead of its preferred source of energy: glucose. This dietary change can be stressful for the body, which may respond by increasing cortisol production. Cortisol is often referred to as the "stress hormone" because its levels rise in response to physical or psychological stress. Therefore, the initial transition to a ketogenic diet can result in elevated cortisol levels in the short term.

However, it's important to note that these changes are usually temporary, and cortisol levels typically normalize as the body adapts to the new diet. Some studies have shown that long-term adherence to a ketogenic diet does not result in chronically elevated cortisol levels.

Other hormonal changes on a ketogenic diet can include changes in thyroid hormones. Some research indicates that a very low-carbohydrate diet like the ketogenic diet may decrease levels of the thyroid hormone T3 and increase reverse T3, which could potentially slow metabolism4. However, more research is needed in this area.

Long-term effects of a ketogenic diet can be beneficial, like improved insulin sensitivity, potentially aiding in weight loss and management of Type 2 diabetes. However, some changes like elevated cortisol levels or altered thyroid hormones may require monitoring. The diet might also lead to nutrient deficiencies if not well-managed. As individual responses can vary greatly, it's crucial to seek professional guidance when considering a major dietary change like the ketogenic diet. Medical or nutritional experts can help ensure the diet is followed safely and is tailored to individual health needs and goals.

Impact of the Ketogenic Diet on Brain Function

As we already know, our brain primarily uses ketones as a source of energy when glucose is low, especially at times of ketogenic diet. Ketones are produced by the liver when it breaks down fats. These ketones are then transported to the brain where they will be converted to molecules that enter the Krebs Cycle to produce energy.

It's interesting to know that such a process takes place and what's even more interesting is that there are more benefits these ketones can bring to our brain than merely as a source of energy. To date, there are already several researches on using the ketogenic diet for the management of various neurological disorders. We will tackle these neurological disorders one by one in the following chapters.

While the exact mechanisms behind these effects are still under investigation, it is believed that the neuroprotective effects of ketones may be due to their ability to reduce inflammation, enhance mitochondrial function, and stimulate the production of neurotrophic factors, proteins that support neuronal survival and function.

In addition, it is suspected that the ketogenic diet not only limits its benefits in managing neurological disorders but extends to enhancing cognitive performance and memory even in healthy individuals. It is also equally compelling to explore other impacts that the ketogenic diet can bring to our brains including mood stability, reduced depression, and behavior improvements.

Overall, the emerging evidence connecting the ketogenic diet to brain health underscores the vital role of nutrition in supporting cognitive function and mental well-being, highlighting the need for further research in this exciting area. It is also important to consult your healthcare provider before you start on a ketogenic diet.

Adding Fiber to the Ketogenic Diet

It is evident that the ketogenic diet has potential benefits for brain health, but what about adding fiber to the mix? Adding fiber to a keto diet can increase its potential health benefits and reduce any risks associated with it.

You can reap several benefits from adding fiber to your diet. First off, fiber can aid your digestion by adding bulk to your stools, promoting regular bowel movement, and preventing constipation. Additionally, fiber-rich foods control hunger because they are more filling compared to the other food groups thus helping you maintain a healthy weight. It is also believed that fiber can lower the risk of developing Type 2 Diabetes and heart diseases, owing to its ability to control blood sugar levels and reduce cholesterol.

Fiber-rich foods are also beneficial to your gut microbiota since they act as prebiotics that provide nourishment to your gut bacteria. A healthy gut microbiota leads to an overall healthy well-being.

Ultimately, fiber doesn't contain too many calories because it is a carbohydrate that your body won't be able to digest.

Thus, it is not easily broken down into sugar molecules, unlike carbohydrates. This makes fiber-rich foods an excellent choice for those aiming to maintain or lose weight, as they can help you feel full without overloading on calories.

Types of Fiber

There are 2 types of fiber; soluble and insoluble. Let us look closely at the difference between these 2 types of fiber.

Soluble Fiber

Soluble fiber is a type of fiber that absorbs water during digestion producing gel-like materials. This helps in slowing down digestion and breaking down carbohydrates slowly into glucose resulting in a regulated glucose in the blood, beneficial to individuals with type 2 diabetes.

Additionally, soluble fiber has been linked with lower levels of low-density lipoprotein (LDL) cholesterol, often referred to as "bad cholesterol." This is because soluble fiber interferes with the absorption of dietary cholesterol, helping to reduce total cholesterol levels in the body. Therefore, incorporating foods high in soluble fiber into your diet can be a great way to improve heart health and support blood sugar management.

Sources of Soluble Fiber:

- Kidney Beans
- Broccoli

- Avocados
- Turnips
- Black Beans
- Lima Beans
- Brussels Sprouts
- Carrots
- Flax Seeds
- Sunflower Seeds
- Guavas
- Apples
- Apricots
- Sweet Potatoes
- Pears
- Figs
- Oats
- Hazelnuts
- Barley
- Psyllium
- Peas
- Citrus Fruits

Insoluble Fiber

Insoluble fiber is a type of dietary fiber that does not dissolve in water. Its primary role is promoting the movement of material through your digestive system and increasing stool bulk, so it can be especially helpful to those who struggle with constipation or irregular stools.

By adding bulk to the stool, insoluble fiber helps prevent constipation and maintain regular bowel movements. This can contribute to digestive health and reduce the risk of developing hemorrhoids and small pouches in your colon (diverticular disease).

Sources of Insoluble Fiber:

- Whole-wheat flour
- Wheat bran
- Nuts
- Artichokes
- Almond
- Cucumbers
- Cauliflower
- Legumes
- Quinoa
- Potatoes
- Leafy Greens

Highly Recommended Fiber Sources

Here are our top choices of fiber sources that can be incorporated into your Ketogenic Diet:

Vegetables

Broccoli: This vegetable is not only rich in fiber but also packed with vitamins C and K. It's great for digestion and provides antioxidants that protect against disease.

Cauliflower: A versatile vegetable, cauliflower is a fantastic source of fiber and can be used as a substitute for rice, mashed potatoes, or even pizza crust.

Spinach: This leafy green is shallow in carbs and high in fiber. It's also an excellent source of several vital vitamins and minerals including iron and calcium.

Fruits

Berries: Most berries are lower in carbs than other fruits and packed with fiber. Raspberries and blackberries contain the most fiber among berries.

Avocados: Although technically a fruit, avocados are often thought of as a vegetable. They're incredibly high in fiber and healthy fats, making them perfect for a ketogenic diet.

Nuts and Seeds

Almonds: Almonds are low in carbs and high in fiber. They're also a good source of protein and healthy fats.

Flax Seeds: Flax seeds are a powerhouse of nutrients. They're packed with fiber and are a great source of omega-3 fatty acids.

Chia Seeds: Chia seeds are one of the best sources of fiber around. They can absorb up to 10 times their weight in water, which helps you feel full and satisfied.

Avocados

Avocados deserve a special mention when talking about a ketogenic diet. They're one of the few fruits that are high in healthy fats and low in carbs. Moreover, they're an excellent source of fiber. A single avocado can provide up to 40% of the daily fiber requirement, making it a staple in many ketogenic diets.

Including these foods in your ketogenic diet can help ensure you're getting enough fiber, while still keeping your carb intake low.

5-Step Guide to Incorporating More Fiber into Your Ketogenic Diet

Adding fiber to your ketogenic diet shouldn't be hard. Here is a comprehensive step-by-step guide that you may follow to incorporate fiber-riched foods into your diet.

Step 1: Choose High isFiber Foods with Low Carbohydrates

Although fiber is generally low in carbohydrates, it is best to choose the lowest of them all with higher fiber content. This is to ensure that your carb intake is controlled and you get the highest fiber possible from your meal. You can take a look back at our top choices of fiber sources as your guide.

Step 2: Gradually Increase your Fiber Intake

If you're new to adding fiber to your meals, it is best that you gradually increase the portion size to give your digestive system time to adjust and avoid digestive discomfort. It is also recommended to add one fiber food at a time to identify what causes the discomfort if there's any, especially if you haven't eaten that fiber source before. For example, you may try sprinkling chia seeds on your salad and if you feel fine after a few hours or days, you can add another fiber-rich food. Repeat these steps until you have reached your desired fiber intake.

Step 3: Stay Hydrated

As you increase your fiber intake, it is also important to increase your water consumption. This is because water is crucial for digestion specifically for breaking down the nutrients from foods so your body can absorb them. Drinking enough water will also prevent constipation and digestive discomfort.

So, how much water should you drink in a day? This is dependent on your fiber intake, the intensity of your physical activity, and the climate you're living in. Normally, the recommended water intake for adults should be eight 8-ounce glasses of water a day. But with high fiber intake and other conditions recently mentioned, you should be drinking more than the recommended volume of water intake in a day.

You can also include other fluids to stay hydrated including herbal tea, soup, and high water content fruits and vegetables.

Ultimately, to reap the benefits of fiber effectively, it is important to increase your fluid intake.

Step 4: Get Creative with Meal Planning

Adding fiber to your diet doesn't have to be boring as there are plenty of ways to make it fun. Stay tuned for our included sample recipes in the following chapters. We'll get creative in turning a humble vegetable or fruit into a healthy, delectable, and enjoyable meal.

Step 5: Consider Adding Fiber Supplements

Fiber supplements can be a helpful addition to your diet if you're finding it difficult to meet your fiber needs through food alone. They come in various forms, including powders, capsules, and chewables, and can be a convenient way to increase your fiber intake.

However, it's important to note that fiber supplements should not replace whole foods. Real foods are complex, offering not just fiber but a wide range of essential nutrients that your body needs. Supplements are meant to "supplement" your diet, not replace parts of it.

Consider these things when looking for fiber supplements:

- *No added sugar*: When looking for a fiber supplement, be sure to check if it has no sugar added. You don't want to add unwanted calories and carbs to your ketogenic diet. Remember that calories and carbs will hinder your body from achieving ketosis.
- *Type of fiber*: There are two types of fiber with two different purposes. There is the soluble fiber that is soluble in water and helps regulate blood glucose and cholesterol. While insoluble fiber does not dissolve in water and is best for aiding other foods to move through your digestive system, promoting regularity.
- *Dosage*: It is recommended to follow the recommended dosage on the back of your fiber supplement for the best result. If it requires you to start with a low dose and then work your way up, better adhere to it. Or consult your general practitioner or licensed dietitian for comprehensive guidance regarding your fiber supplement intake.
- *Water intake*: Always remember that as your fiber intake increases, you should also increase your water consumption. This is because for fiber to work effectively, it needs water and water is very crucial for the digestion process.

So there you have it. Our comprehensive 5-step guide to incorporating fiber-rich foods into your ketogenic diet. Always remember to listen to your body while following these steps. It is also best to consult your doctor or your dietitian before starting a diet or adding supplements to your regimen.

Health Benefits and Use Cases of a High-Fiber Ketogenic Diet

Adding a significant amount of fiber-rich foods to your ketogenic diet has a lot of potential benefits to your overall well-being. Here are some of the benefits of a high-fiber ketogenic diet:

Weight Loss and Management

We already know that the ketogenic diet is an efficient way of managing your weight because it requires less carbohydrate intake to achieve a metabolic state known as ketosis. While in the state of ketosis, your body becomes efficient in burning your fats to be used as an energy source. This alone can help reduce weight and adding high-fiber foods will enhance the effect of the ketogenic diet in managing your weight. High-fiber foods will make you feel full and they have minimal carbohydrate content. This will significantly reduce your hunger and control your calorie intake. Thus, a high-fiber ketogenic diet is an effective diet for weight loss and management.

Improved Digestion and Gut Health

Since fiber adds bulk to the stool, it is very beneficial to healthy digestion and regular bowel movement. Some fiber also acts as a prebiotic, a bacteria that is known to be beneficial to your gut microbiota. This bacteria helps to improve digestion and plays a vital role in the immune function of the body.

Reduced Risk of Heart Disease and Type 2 Diabetes

High-fiber diets have been linked to a reduced risk of heart disease and diabetes. Soluble fiber, in particular, has been shown to lower levels of "bad" LDL cholesterol and regulate blood sugar levels, both of which are key factors in these diseases. The ketogenic diet is also known for its potential to improve insulin sensitivity, further contributing to diabetes prevention and management.

Increased Satiety and Reduced Cravings

As mentioned earlier, fiber-rich foods tend to be more filling than their low-fiber counterparts. This increased satiety can lead to reduced food cravings and less overeating, making it easier to stick to your diet and avoid unhealthy food choices. Moreover, a ketogenic diet can help stabilize blood sugar levels, which can also help control cravings.

Enhanced Mental Clarity and Energy Levels

The ketogenic diet is known to improve neurological health because ketones, the byproduct of ketosis, are a more efficient fuel source for the brain compared to glucose. Thus, a ketogenic diet incorporated with high-fiber foods is beneficial to an individual's mental well-being.

Reduced Inflammation

Both the ketogenic diet and high fiber intake have been linked to reduced inflammation in the body. Chronic inflammation is associated with many serious diseases, including heart disease, cancer, and Alzheimer's. By reducing inflammation, a high-fiber ketogenic diet could potentially contribute to the prevention of these conditions.

Improved Skin Health

There are a lot of factors that come into play as to why a high-fiber ketogenic diet can improve your skin health. The first reason is a ketogenic diet requires a low carbohydrate intake that would result in reduced calories and insulin. It is thought that a high level of insulin in the body can lead to inflammation that causes acne and other skin flaws. Another reason why a high-fiber ketogenic diet is beneficial for skin health is that the ketones produced during ketosis have anti-inflammatory properties. In addition, fiber-rich foods are beneficial for gut health. A healthy gut microbiota is believed to have an impact on skin conditions.

In conclusion, a high-fiber ketogenic diet could potentially improve skin health by reducing inflammation and supporting gut health. However, more research is needed in this area, and individual responses may vary.

Women and the Ketogenic Diet

In this chapter, we'll discuss the unique relationship between women and the ketogenic diet. We will elaborate on the unique needs of women in terms of nutrients compared to men as well as the effect of the ketogenic diet specifically for women. We'll also talk about the potential drawbacks of this diet and the things to take note of before getting started with the ketogenic diet.

How Women's Nutritional Needs Differ from Men's

Men and women have different nutritional requirements due to physiological differences, including hormonal fluctuations and body composition. This section will examine these differences in detail, highlighting why a one-size-fits-all approach to nutrition does not work.

Hormonal Differences

Women's menstrual cycle has a bigger impact on their nutritional needs. There are two primary phases of a woman's menstrual cycle: the pre-ovulation phase or the follicular phase and the post-ovulation phase also known as the luteal phase. During these phases, women's nutritional needs vary.

For instance, during the pre-ovulation phase, there is a notable rise in the estrogen level. This hormone is responsible for the decrease in women's blood sugar levels as it has been linked to the body's increased ability to process carbohydrates.

While during the post-ovulation phase, estrogen and progesterone are both at high levels. Progesterone has been linked to an increase in appetite and cravings for high-fat and sugary foods. In this phase, women may experience increased caloric needs because of the increase in the metabolic rate.

Moreover, fluctuations in hormones can also affect water retention and digestion, further influencing a woman's nutritional needs and metabolism throughout her menstrual cycle. For example, some women may experience bloating or constipation due to hormonal changes, which could be alleviated by increasing the intake of dietary fiber and fluids.

Therefore, while following a ketogenic diet, women should consider these hormonal changes and adjust their diet according to their body's signals and needs, especially during different phases of their menstrual cycle. This might mean slightly increasing carbohydrate intake during the follicular phase or ensuring adequate caloric intake during the luteal phase.

Iron Requirements

During menstruation, women lose about 30-40 milligrams of iron per cycle on average. It is important to note that during this stage, it is best to compensate for the Iron loss to avoid Iron deficiency that causes anemia.

For women following a ketogenic diet, it's important to ensure they're consuming enough iron-rich foods. While meat and seafood are good sources of iron, those on a vegetarian or vegan ketogenic diet can turn to iron-rich vegetables like spinach and broccoli, or seeds and nuts. Pairing these foods with a source of vitamin C can enhance iron absorption. However, considering the restrictive nature of a ketogenic diet, some women might need to consider an iron supplement under medical supervision.

Calcium and Vitamin D

Compared to men, women are at higher risk for osteoporosis, especially during menopause. Estrogen is also responsible for keeping the bone healthy by protecting it against bone loss. During menopause, there is a rapid decrease in estrogen levels in women which often leads to osteoporosis. Understanding the effect of this hormone on women's bone health will give light to the importance of adding Calcium and Vitamin D-rich foods or supplements to the ketogenic diet. Good sources of Vitamin D and Calcium include leafy green vegetables and fish. However, with the restrictive nature of the ketogenic diet, women following this diet may opt for supplements with proper medical supervision.

Caloric Needs

It is known that men require more caloric intake compared to women. This is owing to the differences in muscle mass, activities, and body size and composition. The estimated caloric intake for women is between 1,600 - 2,400 while men require 2,000 - 3,000 calories per day. However, these estimates may vary across all individuals.

For women following the ketogenic diet for weight loss, it is important to note that you still need to monitor your caloric intake since extra calories in the body will lead to weight gain regardless if it comes from carbohydrates, fats, or proteins.

As always, it's recommended to consult with a healthcare provider or a registered dietitian to determine individual caloric needs, especially when following a specific diet plan like the ketogenic diet.

Benefits of the Ketogenic Diet Specifically for Women

The ketogenic diet offers several benefits to women including hormonal balance, weight management, and healthy skin. In this chapter, we'll dive deep into the benefits of the ketogenic diet to women.

Weight loss

Several factors aid weight loss while on a ketogenic diet:

- *Suppressed Appetite*: Ketogenic diets tend to be quite filling due to their high protein and fat content, which can lead to reduced calorie intake.
- *Increased Fat Burning*: In ketosis, your body uses fat as its primary source of fuel, which can increase fat burning.
- *Lower Insulin Levels*: By reducing carbohydrates, ketogenic diets can lower insulin levels, making it easier for your body to access and burn stored fat.
- *Water Weight Loss*: Initially, the ketogenic diet can result in rapid weight loss as the body depletes its glycogen stores and secretes bound water.

These factors might be beneficial to obese women who are struggling to lose their weight. However, it is still best to consult a doctor or professional dietitian before following any diet.

Hormonal Balance

The most common hormonal disorder in women is Polycystic Ovary Syndrome or PCOS. This hormonal disorder is often associated with irregular menstrual cycles, excess hair growth, acne, and obesity. While the exact cause of PCOS has not been pinpointed yet, it is often linked to insulin resistance.

The ketogenic diet is known to aid insulin sensitivity and promote weight loss which may help women with PCOS for the following reasons:

- *Insulin Sensitivity*: High levels of insulin have been linked to stimulating the ovary to produce male hormones that cause hormonal imbalance. The ketogenic diet controls the insulin level in your body and may help the ovary produce male hormones and manage PCOS syndromes.
- *Weight loss*: Women with PCOS are commonly challenged with their weight management. The ketogenic diet promotes weight loss thereby beneficial to women with PCOS.

While these factors may help alleviate the symptoms of PCOS, it is important to note that it shouldn't be used as an alternative cure for this disorder. It is still best to consult your Obgyne for guided meditation.

Heart Health

As previously discussed, the ketogenic diet is beneficial in lowering the body's bad cholesterol that causes heart disease. It also promotes weight loss which is beneficial to your heart health since obesity has been linked to one of the risk factors for heart disease. Additionally, a low-carb diet may help lower the blood pressure.

For women, especially post-menopause when the risk of heart disease increases due to the decrease in protective estrogen levels, it's crucial to approach a ketogenic diet with caution and under the guidance of a healthcare provider.

Skin Health

The ketogenic diet could potentially improve skin health in women by reducing inflammation and oxidative stress, aiding collagen production, and decreasing acne breakouts. However, individual responses may vary, and some may initially experience skin issues. Always consult a healthcare provider before starting a new diet.

Precautions and Potential Side Effects for Women on a Ketogenic Diet

While the ketogenic diet can be beneficial, women must be aware of potential side effects and considerations. This part of the chapter will outline the precautions women should take when embarking on a ketogenic diet and discuss the potential side effects they may encounter.

- *Nutrient Deficiencies*: Since the ketogenic diet is a food-restrictive diet, there are potential nutrient deficiencies for individuals following this diet. Thus, it is important to take note of the nutritional needs that we previously discussed to prevent nutrient deficiencies while on this diet.

- *Menstrual Cycle and Fertility*: Some women may experience irregularity in their menstrual cycle due to a drastic change in diet. Always consult a specialist or professional dietitian before following any diet.
- *Bone Health*: Remember to take into consideration incorporating foods that are high in calcium and vitamin D while on a ketogenic diet. However, since this diet is restrictive and may cause nutrient deficiency, it is recommended to take supplements for your bone health while following this diet.
- *Keto Flu*: At some early stage of starting this diet, advocates may feel flu-like symptoms including fatigue, headache, and irritability. This is just your body adjusting to your diet changes. Always consult your professional dietitian for proper guidance.
- *Importance of Medical Supervision*: Given these potential risks, women must undertake a ketogenic diet under medical supervision to ensure they're meeting nutritional needs and monitoring any changes in health.

Women and Fiber

Fiber plays a crucial role in women's health. It aids in digestion, helps maintain a healthy weight, lowers the risk of diabetes and heart disease, and can even reduce the risk of certain types of cancer, such as breast cancer.

Unique Benefits of High-Fiber Diets for Women

A high-fiber diet offers unique benefits for women. For instance, it can help manage hormonal imbalances by binding to excess estrogen in the digestive tract and removing it from the body. It also aids in weight management, a concern for many women, especially during menopause when metabolism slows down. A high-fiber diet can also promote healthier skin by moving yeast and fungus out of the body, preventing them from being excreted through the skin where they can trigger acne or rashes.

Recommended Daily Fiber Intake for Women

The American Heart Association recommends at least 25 grams of fiber per day for women under 50, and 21 grams per day for women over 50. However, the average American woman only consumes about half of the recommended amount. To increase fiber intake, women should aim to include a variety of fruits, vegetables, whole grains, and legumes in their diets.

Remember, it's essential to increase fiber intake gradually and drink plenty of water to avoid digestive discomfort.

Sample Recipes: High-Fiber Keto Meals for Women

Ketogenic Pizza

Ingredients:

- Crust
- 4 eggs
- 3 oz. shredded cheese, either provolone or mozzarella
- 3 oz. chia seed or flax seeds
- Topping
- 3 tbsp of tomato sauce, unsweetened
- 1 tsp dried oregano
- 5 oz. of cheese, shredded
- 1½ oz. pepperoni
- 1/2 cup of thinly sliced bell peppers
- 1/2 cup mushrooms, sliced
- 1/2 cup spinach, roughly chopped
- 1/2 cup broccoli florets, chopped into small pieces
- 1/4 cup artichokes, canned or marinated, chopped

For serving:

- 2 oz. leafy greens
- 4 tbsp olive oil
- sea salt and ground black pepper
- pumpkin seeds or sunflower seeds

Instructions:

1. Preheat the oven to 400°F (200°C).

2. Start by making the crust. Crack eggs into a medium-sized bowl and add shredded cheese and chia seeds. Give it a good stir to combine.
3. Use a spatula to spread the batter on a baking sheet lined with parchment paper.
4. You can form two circles or just make one large rectangular pizza.
5. Set the pizza in the oven and let it cook for 15 minutes until the crust acquires a golden hue.
6. Remove and let cool for a minute or two.
7. Set the temperature of the oven to 450°F (225°C).
8. Spread tomato sauce on the crust and add the toppings according to your preferences. Let your creativity shine!
9. Bake for another 5-10 minutes or until the pizza has turned a golden brown color.
10. Serve with a fresh salad on the side.

High-Fiber Keto Pesto Chicken

Ingredients:

- 1½ lbs boneless chicken thighs or chicken breasts
- salt and pepper
- 1/2 cup of chopped artichoke hearts
- 2 tbsp butter or coconut oil
- 5 tbsp red pesto or green pesto
- 1¼ cups heavy whipping cream
- 3 oz. pitted olives
- 5 oz. feta cheese, diced
- 1 garlic clove, finely chopped

For serving:

- 5 oz. mixed greens (spinach, kale, arugula)
- 1/4 cup diced cucumber
- 1/4 cup shredded carrots
- 2 tbsp of pumpkin seeds or chia seeds

Dressing:

- olive oil
- sea salt
- black pepper

Instructions:

1. Meanwhile, cut the chicken into bite-sized pieces. Season with salt and pepper.

2. Add butter or oil to a large skillet and fry the chicken pieces in batches on medium-high heat until golden brown.
3. Preheat the oven to 400°F (200°C).
4. Place the fried chicken pieces in a baking dish together with the chopped artichoke hearts, olives, feta cheese, and garlic.
5. Using store-bought low-carb red or green pesto, or making your own, mix pesto and heavy cream in a bowl.
6. Add the pesto/cream mixture.
7. Bake in the oven for 20-30 minutes, until the dish turns bubbly and light brown around the edges.
8. Serve with high-fiber salad when fully cooked.

High-Fiber Ketogenic Mushroom Omelet

Ingredients:

- 4 large mushrooms, sliced
- 3 eggs
- 1/4 cup of chopped spinach
- 1 oz. butter, for frying
- 1 oz. shredded cheese
- ¼ yellow onion, chopped
- 1 tablespoon of flaxseeds or chia seeds
- salt, and pepper

Instructions:

1. Crack the eggs into a mixing bowl with a pinch of salt and pepper.
2. Whisk the eggs with a fork until smooth and frothy.
3. Melt the butter in a frying pan, over medium heat.
4. Add the mushrooms, chopped spinach, and onion to the pan, stirring until tender, and then pour in the egg mixture, surrounding the veggies.
5. When the omelet begins to cook and get firm, but still has a little raw egg on top, sprinkle cheese and chia seeds or flax seeds over the egg.
6. Using a spatula, carefully ease around the edges of the omelet, and then fold it over in half.

7. When it starts to turn golden brown underneath, remove the pan from the heat and slide the omelet onto a plate.

Chicken Pot Pie

Ingredients:

For the chicken filling:

- 1 tablespoon butter
- 1.5 pounds organic chicken breasts, cut into ½ inch cubes
- 4 ounces yellow onion, finely chopped
- ½ cup broccoli
- ¼ cup spinach
- 1 clove garlic, crushed
- ½ teaspoon dried thyme
- 1 tablespoon white wine vinegar
- 1 cup chicken broth, low-sodium
- ¼ cup peas, fresh or frozen (no need to defrost)
- ½ cup coconut cream
- ¼– ½ teaspoon sea salt (taste before adding)
- ¼ teaspoon freshly ground black pepper

For the topping:

- 1 cup superfine almond flour
- 1 tablespoon ground flax seeds
- ½ teaspoon xanthan gum
- 1 teaspoon baking powder
- ¼ teaspoon of sea salt
- 2 tablespoons butter, cut into large chunks
- 2 tablespoons sour cream

- 1 egg white

Instructions:

1. Set the temperature of the oven to 400°F and preheat.
2. Grease a 9" round baking pan.

For the chicken filling:

1. Heat a large skillet over medium-high heat. Melt butter in the skillet.
2. When the butter has melted and is no longer foaming, add the diced chicken to the pan.
3. Cook chicken, stirring occasionally, until chicken begins to brown on all sides, but is not yet cooked throughout.
4. Add onion, broccoli, and spinach to the skillet.
5. Lightly season the mixture with a dash of salt and pepper.
6. Set the heat to medium-low. Keep stirring from time to time until the onions start to show signs of browning at their edges, although they're not fully soft yet.
7. Stir in garlic and dried thyme. Cook for one minute, stirring constantly.
8. Stir in vinegar, scraping up browned bits. When the vinegar has almost completely evaporated, stir in broth.

9. Adjust the heat to medium-high. Stir the broth occasionally, allowing it to condense and thicken over a period of 15-20 minutes.
10. Season to taste with salt and pepper, if necessary.
11. Turn the heat to low. Simmer until the mixture is thick and gravy-like. Taste before adding salt and pepper.
12. Once the broth has thickened, add coconut cream and peas. Bring mixture to a simmer.
13. While the filling simmers, prepare the biscuit topping.
14. The broth is thick enough that you can "draw" a line on the bottom of the pan with a spoon, and the line does not immediately fill in.

For the topping:

1. In a mixing bowl, mix together the almond flour, xanthan gum, ground flax seeds, baking powder, and salt.
2. Mix the butter into the dry ingredients using a pastry blender. The mixture should appear mealy.
3. In a small bowl, whisk the sour cream and the egg whites together.
4. Stir this mixture into the dry ingredients.
5. Gather the mixture into a ball and place it on a piece of parchment paper or a counter dusted with almond flour.

6. Using clean hands or a rolling pin dusted with almond flour, press or roll dough into a circle about 8 inches in diameter.

To assemble:

1. Pour chicken filling into the prepared baking dish.
2. Gently place biscuit dough over the chicken filling.
3. Bake in a preheated oven for 10-12 minutes, or until the biscuit topping has been browned.

Avocado and Chicken Salad with Lemon Vinaigrette

Ingredients:

- 2 cups cooked chicken breast, shredded
- 1 ripe avocado, diced
- 1 cup cucumber, diced
- ½ cup cherry tomatoes, halved
- ¼ cup red onion, thinly sliced
- 2 tablespoons chopped fresh cilantro
- Juice of 1 lemon
- 2 tablespoons extra virgin olive oil
- Salt and pepper to taste
- 4 cups mixed greens

Instructions:

1. In a large bowl, combine the shredded chicken, diced avocado, cucumber, cherry tomatoes, red onion, and cilantro.
2. In a small bowl, whisk together the lemon juice, olive oil, salt, and pepper to make the vinaigrette.
3. Pour the vinaigrette over the chicken and avocado mixture. Toss gently to coat everything evenly.
4. Divide the mixed greens onto four plates.
5. Spoon the avocado and chicken salad over the greens, distributing it evenly.
6. Serve immediately and enjoy!

Cheesy Taco Skillet with Cauliflower Rice

Ingredients:

- 1 lb ground beef
- 1/4 medium onion diced
- 1/2 red pepper diced
- 3 tbsp taco seasoning
- 1 cup diced tomatoes
- 12 ounces cauliflower rice fresh or frozen
- 1/2 cup chicken broth
- 1 1/2 cups shredded Cheddar cheese or Mexican Blend

Instructions:

1. In a large skillet over medium heat, brown the ground beef until almost cooked through (just a little pink).
2. Add the onion and pepper and continue to cook until no longer pink.
3. Stir in the taco seasoning.
4. Add the tomatoes and cauliflower rice and stir to combine. Stir in the broth and bring to a simmer.
5. Reduce the heat to medium-low and cook until the cauliflower rice begins to soften (8 to 10 minutes for frozen).
6. Sprinkle the skillet with the cheese and cover.
7. Let cook until the cheese is melted, 3 or 4 minutes.

8. Take it off the heat and garnish with your preferred toppings such as avocado, sour cream, and freshly chopped cilantro.

Western Omelet

Ingredients:

- 6 eggs
- 2 tbsp heavy whipping cream or sour cream
- salt and pepper
- 3 oz. shredded cheese, divided
- 2 oz. butter
- 5 oz. smoked deli ham, diced
- ½ yellow onion, finely chopped
- ½ green bell pepper, finely chopped
- 1 cup chopped spinach
- ¼ cup sliced mushroom

Instructions:

1. In a mixing bowl, whisk eggs and cream until fluffy.
2. Add salt and pepper.
3. Add half of the shredded cheese and mix well.
4. Melt the butter in a large frying pan on medium heat.
5. Sauté the diced ham, onion, spinach, mushroom, and peppers for a few minutes.
6. Add the egg mixture and fry until the omelet is almost firm. Be extra mindful not to burn the edges.
7. Reduce the heat after a little while. Sprinkle the rest of the cheese on top and fold the omelet.
8. Cut the omelet in half, serve immediately... and enjoy!

Conclusion

Congratulations on completing this whole guide about the high-fiber ketogenic diet. You may have concluded this reading, but your journey toward mental, dermatological, and overall health starts here. It may be a long and bumpy journey but a healthy eating habit will always be worth it in the end.

Always watch out and listen to your body though. Take note of how your body reacts to every new food or meal that you eat. Start slow and work your way up toward your health goals. If ever you experience setbacks, always remember that you're making progress. Just pick up where you left off and take a step forward at a time.

Disclaimer: This guide is for educational purposes only and should not be used as a substitute for professional advice. It is always best to consult your general practitioner or professional dietitian.

FAQ

What Is a Ketogenic Diet?

A ketogenic diet is a high-fat, low-carbohydrate diet that is effective in promoting weight loss and improving health. The goal of the diet is to put your body into a state of ketosis, which occurs when your body starts burning fat for energy instead of carbohydrates. This can lead to rapid weight loss, improved blood sugar control, and increased energy levels.

What Are the Benefits of Following a Ketogenic Diet?

Research has shown that following a ketogenic diet can have numerous benefits, including improved blood sugar control, increased energy levels, and rapid weight loss. Additionally, the diet has been linked to improved brain health and cognitive function as well as reduced inflammation in the body.

How Much Fiber Should I Eat on a Ketogenic Diet?

The amount of fiber you should eat on a ketogenic diet depends on your individual needs and goals. Generally speaking, it is recommended that you consume 25-35 grams of fiber per day while following a ketogenic diet. It is important to note that some sources of fiber may be higher in carbohydrates than others so it's important to read labels carefully when selecting foods with fiber.

What Foods Can I Eat on a Ketogenic Diet?

When following a ketogenic diet it's important to focus on consuming high-quality fats such as olive oil, avocado oil, coconut oil, nuts, and seeds as well as plenty of non-starchy vegetables such as leafy greens and cruciferous vegetables like broccoli and cauliflower. Protein sources should include fatty fish such as salmon or tuna as well as grass-fed meats such as beef or lamb.

Are There Any Risks Associated With Following A High-Fiber Ketogenic Diet?

Yes - if not done correctly there are potential risks associated with following any type of restrictive eating plan including nutrient deficiencies due to inadequate intake of certain vitamins or minerals or an imbalance between macronutrients (carbs/fats/protein). Therefore it's important to speak with your doctor before starting any new nutrition program or making drastic changes to your current eating habits.

Are There Any Special Considerations For Women When Following A High Fiber Ketogenic Diet?

Yes - women have different nutritional needs than men due to hormonal fluctuations throughout their lifetime so it's important for them to pay special attention when choosing foods for their high-fiber keto meal plan to ensure they are getting adequate amounts of key nutrients such as iron, calcium, and vitamin D for optimal health outcomes.

References and Helpful Links

Metamucil. (2023). How to get fiber on keto. www.metamucil.com. https://www.metamucil.com/en-us/articles/fiber-supplements/how-to-sup plement-your-lack-of-fiber-on-the-keto-diet

Cissn, R. M. M. (2023, June 28). The Ketogenic Diet: A detailed beginner's guide to keto. Healthline. https://www.healthline.com/nutrition/ketogenic-diet-101

Eenfeldt, A., MD, & Scher, B., MD. (2022, November 29). A ketogenic diet for beginners. Diet Doctor. https://www.dietdoctor.com/low-carb/keto

Holloway, C. (2023, August 3). 31 High-Fiber foods you should be eating. Cleveland Clinic. https://health.clevelandclinic.org/high-fiber-foods/

De Bellefonds, C., Miller, K., & Lam, J. (2023, September 26). 40 High-Fiber Foods That Should Be On Your Plate Every Day, According To Nutritionists. Women's Health. https://www.womenshealthmag.com/food/a19967218/foods-high-in-fiber /

Brighten, J. (2022). Keto for Women: the risks, benefits, and how it impacts hormones. Dr. Jolene Brighten. https://drbrighten.com/keto-and-womens-health/

Gottfried, S., MD. (2021, September 21). Women, food, and hormones: Why keto doesn't work for all women - Sara Gottfried MD. Sara Gottfried MD. https://www.saragottfriedmd.com/women-food-and-hormones-why-keto-doesnt-work-for-all-women/